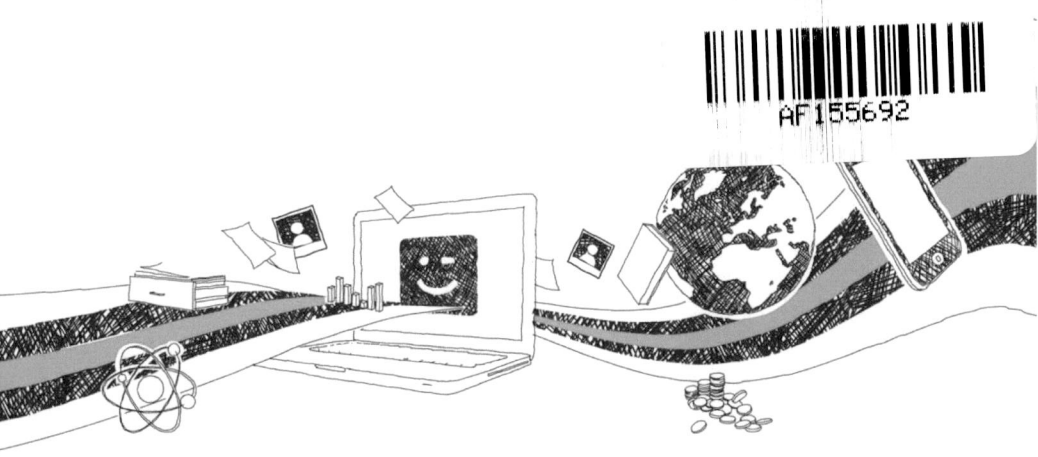
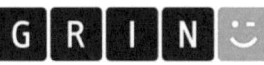

Bibliographic information published by the German National Library:

The German National Library lists this publication in the National Bibliography; detailed bibliographic data are available on the Internet at http://dnb.dnb.de .

Imprint:

Copyright © 2017 GRIN Verlag, Open Publishing GmbH
Print and binding: Books on Demand GmbH, Norderstedt Germany
ISBN: 9783668470743

This book at GRIN:

http://www.grin.com/en/e-book/369485/emerging-health-care-delivery-models-in-the-us-and-how-they-improve-the

James Mageto

Emerging health care delivery models in the US and how they improve the quality of care

GRIN Publishing

GRIN - Your knowledge has value

Since its foundation in 1998, GRIN has specialized in publishing academic texts by students, college teachers and other academics as e-book and printed book. The website www.grin.com is an ideal platform for presenting term papers, final papers, scientific essays, dissertations and specialist books.

Visit us on the internet:

http://www.grin.com/

http://www.facebook.com/grincom

http://www.twitter.com/grin_com

Annotated Bibliography: Emerging health care delivery models in the US and how they improve

quality of care

Name

Institution

Value-based care: better care, better health, lower costs. (n.d.). The Health System. Retrieved

March 6, 2017

This is a great article that majorly focusses on value-based healthcare delivery model and

it describes what value-based delivery model means and entails and goes further to explain in

details the four types of value-based delivery model, which are Accountable Care Organization

(ACO), Patient-Centered Medical Home(PCMH), Pay for Performance (P4P) and Bundled

Payments. Value-based healthcare delivery model is a solution that is emerging and it aims at

addressing the healthcare costs that keep on rising and to make it cheaper and easier for people to

find the care they need. In this model, hospitals and their doctors get payments for keeping

people healthy and for ensuring the health of chronic diseases patients gets to improve in an

evidence-based approach and a cost effective manner. The article further explains that this value-

based model is designed around and for patients, who in the end benefit from a team concerned

with coordination of their health and give the correct information to help them get the right care

across our healthcare system. All individual patient needs are met by the medical care teams

whether they be chronic, acute or preventive. The article concludes that whatever the value-

based model you choose, all of them aim at delivering better health in a more affordable way.

Moreover, the way a value-based care will look depends on what approach the doctors and

healthcare systems take in its implementation. Some of the models are very visible while others

are invisible and therefore you may get care under one of these models and never even know that

you have. I therefore find this article very descriptive on my topic of interest and is gives very

vital information that I need for my research paper.

The Medical Home Model of Care. (september 2012). Health. Retrieved March 6, 2017, from

    http://www.ncsl.org/research/health/the-medical-home-model-of-care.aspx

    This article is authored by the National Conference of State Legislatures and was last updated in September 2012 meaning it is up to date and contains information that can be relied on. It focusses majorly on the Medical Home Model of healthcare that offers one method of transforming the healthcare delivery system. It further explains that medical homes can lower costs while improving on the efficiency and quality of the healthcare services via an innovative approach in delivering a comprehensive and patient-oriented medical care. It is also called the Patient-Centered Medical Home (PCMH) and is designed to meet patient needs and its aim is improving patient access to medical care e.g. through extension of office hours and increased communication between patients and medical care providers via telephone and mail, increase coordination in medical care and enhance overall medical care quality. All these should happen while at the same time reducing costs. PCMH relies on a team of medical care providers such as nurses, pharmacists, and physicians, who are tasked to meet all the healthcare needs of their patients. The article further explains that from the various researches and studies that have been done, they show that medical home improves both physical and behavioral health, access to social services that are community based and chronic conditions management. Since the article has been authored by a state agency that has done intense research on the topic presented here, I can rely on it to form part of the content of my paper as the source is reliable. Therefore, this article will be of great help and importance to me in writing my research paper.

Davis, J. R. (2000). Managed care systems and emerging infections: challenges and opportunities

    for strengthening research, surveillance and prevention: workshop summary.

    Washington, D.C.: National Academy Press. Retrieved March 5, 2017.

The author of this book has done a thorough research and study on managed health care delivery and came to find out that as the health care systems of the nation keep on evolving and are being restructured, the managed care organizations are most likely to cause major effects both on health care delivery and also other aspects of public health. For instance, these organizations have a high potential of spearheading the fight against diseases which are infectious in terms of research, prevention and treatment and this is likely to bring huge improvements in the health status of the community at large. The author also found out that in as much as the managed health care organizations have so many benefits to people, they can be a barrier to efficient collaboration between the public health society and the managed care organizations, if reimbursements of expenditures in health care are not considered well and carefully. This book presents a well-structured research content on health care and an in-depth explanation and health care history in the nation. He has explained what health care organizations are, given the various types of these organizations and even gone further to explain the benefits and advantages of these health care organizations. This book is therefore quite useful for my research in that it provides an in-depth explanation on health care systems. Besides, based on the authors' credentials, the book is reliable and can be depended upon. The author is a prolific researcher and therefore, I find the book very useful, and reliable.

A. P., Director of Business Development, VitalHealth Software. (april 25, 2013). Getting ready
     for emerging care models. Retrieved March 5, 2017.

This article has been written by Andrew Pashman, who is the business development
director at VitalHealth Software, a developer of software for management of health which is
cloud-based. The company majorly focuses on management of diseases, management of health
network and management of personal health and was founded as a collaboration between the
Mayo Clinic and Noaber Foundation. Currently, physicians are involved in the preparations
towards the participation in the value-based care delivery models such as PCMHs, ACOs and
networks that are clinically integrated. The preparations can be categorized into three areas
namely: processes, people and technology. This article majorly focusses on the foundational
technology layer that is required in order to take part in these new health delivery models.
According to this article, for you to take part in a value-based delivery model, you have to be
willing and able to collaborate and coordinate on patient care with other outpatient providers.
The goal of value-based delivery models is to provide the right and required amount of
preventive care, to avoid complications in health and to give better patient care which has lower
attendant costs. The article therefore finds great use for my research topic for the information
provided will help develop content for my research topic. Moreover, the article was published 3
years ago, and that makes it quite valid, and updated, meaning that it bears usable information to
my research topic.

J. S., Partner, Access Market Intelligence, Greenville, SC, & F. V., Partner, Access Market

Intelligence, Greenville, SC, Adjunct Professor of Pharmacy Administration,

Presbyterian College School of Pharmacy, Clinton, SC, and Adjunct Instructor,

Outcomes and Health Policy, University of Illinois at Chicago College of Pharmacy.

(2015 feb). Key Strategic Trends that Impact Healthcare Decision-Making and

Stakeholder Roles in the New Marketplace. 15-20. Retrieved March 5, 2017.

This article describes the effect of change and its impact on the stakeholders in the

healthcare sector from 2010 to date and the passage of reforms in healthcare in the United States.

Despite the fact that most of the early changes in healthcare market have widely been published,

emerging trends at the national level require identification for the healthcare market to succeed.

Those high-level trends that will be identified affect decision-making and healthcare roles and

they have the ability to transform the healthcare market and affect relationships between various

stakeholders. This articles goes further to explain that business or personal consequences that are

related to these trends are very important as they will keep all stakeholders aware of their

impacts and therefore be able to prepare for their impact. Therefore, individual stakeholders have

to innovate and/or adapt to these trends and they will also need to understand their impact on

clinical care decision-making. The clinical care decisions which are shared among the various

stakeholders will need to balance both clinical consequences and economic aspects among the

various stakeholders. This new reality will not be avoidable in oncology care as it already exists

there and it is difficult to change. The article concludes that for all the healthcare stakeholders to

be prepared well, they need to be aware of early tracing as well as of the various trends that keep

on emerging in the healthcare sector. I therefore find this article very crucial and reliable in my topic of research as it is elaborative, vivid and very clear in its content that has been well researched and structured.

References

J. S., Partner, Access Market Intelligence, Greenville, SC, & F. V., Partner, Access Market

    Intelligence, Greenville, SC, Adjunct Professor of Pharmacy Administration,

    Presbyterian College School of Pharmacy, Clinton, SC, and Adjunct Instructor,

    Outcomes and Health Policy, University of Illinois at Chicago College of Pharmacy.

    (2015 feb). Key Strategic Trends that Impact Healthcare Decision-Making and

    Stakeholder Roles in the New Marketplace. 15-20. Retrieved March 5, 2017.

Davis, J. R. (2000). Managed care systems and emerging infections: challenges and opportunities

    for strengthening research, surveillance and prevention: workshop summary.

    Washington, D.C.: National Academy Press. Retrieved March 5, 2017.

A. P., Director of Business Development, VitalHealth Software. (april 25, 2013). Getting ready

    for emerging care models. Retrieved March 5, 2017.

Value-based care: better care, better health, lower costs. (n.d.). The Health System. Retrieved

    March 6, 2017

The Medical Home Model of Care. (september 2012). Health. Retrieved March 6, 2017, from

    http://www.ncsl.org/research/health/the-medical-home-model-of-care.aspx

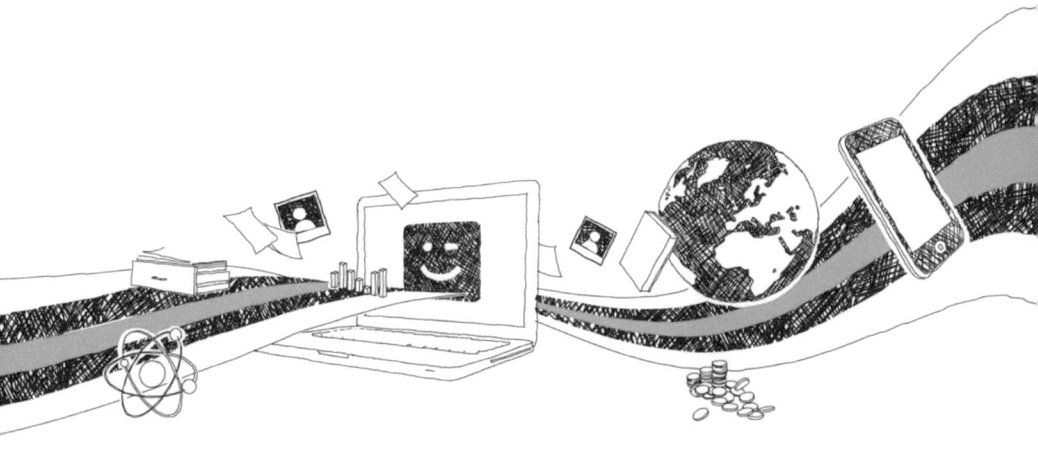
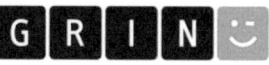